Morning Sickn
Bridie Bell

Morning Sickness

66 life-saving hacks

to help you survive pregnancy-related nausea, vomiting, and reflux

Bridie Bell

Cover by Rudi Hartono.

Book and e-book design by Bulaja naklada, Zagreb

www.busymama.com.au

Contents

Foreword

SWIRLING, SEASICK FEELING from your abdomen up to your throat? Check.

Uncomfortable pressure around your middle? Check.

Pools of saliva welling in the recesses of your mouth? Check.

Compulsive need to yawn, take a deep breath, or close your eyes? Check.

Zero energy? Feelings of misery and despair? Love/hate relationship with food? Check. Check. Check.

Okay, enough! We don't want to make you feel even worse by reminding you of your symptoms! But the point we want to make is that, for many, morning sickness is more than the occasional sensation of nausea first thing in the morning.

I'm a morning sickness survivor. Between two pregnancies I have conquered over 40 relentless weeks of daily nausea and worse. I know exactly how all-consuming it can be. It can be maddening. It can be isolating. I personally remember feeling like there was no joy left in my life. Well, unless I counted the fleeting sense of relief after throwing up! Boy, how my standards had dropped!

And yet I made it! Not only that, I came through to the other side relatively unscathed, with a beautiful boy and a darling girl. When you read my story, you'll see that as painful as morning sickness was, it was all worth it – and the experience of overcoming this hurdle drove me to share my remedies and help other mums.

How did I survive? How did I manage to resuscitate my appetite, recharge my energy, and reawaken my positive feelings about pregnancy?

Well, I did my research. I talked with other women and, above all, I engaged in lots of trial and error. After all (and this is true for you, too), you won't really know if something works until you give it a go for yourself. Amazingly, I found that there *are* things you can do to help your situation. Sometimes the smallest change to your habits can make a huge difference to your everyday experience of morning sickness. The little things really do add up in helping you through.

Like me, you probably just want to find some solutions that work. Sounds simple enough, but at times it seemed almost impossible. I couldn't understand why it was so difficult to find accurate, straightforward information that was easy to digest (pardon the pun!). Of course, there are already plenty of books devoted to morning sickness, and some of them are excellent. But really, when you collapse on your bed after another exhausting session in the bathroom, do you have the energy to plough through an entire novel? I sure didn't! Mama blogs, websites, and forums have snippets of valuable advice, but it is fragmented and incomplete.

From my own experience, I know that suffering through morning sickness can cause extreme emotional stress for a lot of mamas and their families too often. It can feel like an untenable situation. You might be hysterical with tiredness and incapacitated by nausea, but the only person who can help your situation is you.

So, looking back, I wanted to share with you my arsenal of amazing morning sickness hacks – remedies and tips to help you navigate through this time with knowledge and confidence. I based the style of this book on my own need for clear, uncomplicated advice (and the difficulty I had in finding such a resource!). *Morning Sickness – 66 Life-Saving Hacks to help you survive pregnancy-related nausea, vomiting, and reflux* eliminates the need to trawl the internet for piecemeal information. I have taken care of the research for you, and this is the result: a carefully curated list of remedies and hacks.

This book is designed to be read at any stage in your pregnancy, whenever you are feeling any of the sickly effects of our blessed hormones. Above all, I wanted to create a book that is about *action*. That gets straight to the point and offers hope and inspiration. My hope is that by following the advice in this book, you will be able to take charge of improving your wellbeing.

Bridie's story

When I found out I was pregnant, I was thrilled. Years of studying, working, and enjoying my twenties meant that by the time I married 'the one' I was already in my early thirties. So, after a beautiful wedding and indulgently long honeymoon, my husband and I decided to start our family without delay.

I was an avid follower of pregnancy and conception websites. My phone history revealed ridiculously regular visits to forums where hopeful mamas-to-be discussed the early symptoms of pregnancy. I spent enough time lurking around the web to know every possible sign of successful conception, from twinges below the bellybutton to gums bleeding at night. Feelings of morning sickness and aversion to foods and smells seemed to be especially common. Random throwing up. Nausea and light-headedness. Was it possible to have morning sickness before you even tested positive as pregnant? I didn't know. And I honestly didn't care. As far as I was concerned, a bit of nausea was a small price to pay to be part of the mothers--to-be club. For me, morning sickness was almost a romantic notion, the stuff of TV ads and movies. You know how it goes – the woman feels a sudden urge to run out of the room when eating dinner and people immediately give each other knowing looks. There's a baby on the way!

A few months later, my test result was positive – I was pregnant! I clearly remember telling my mum only a week later that I wished I had more signs. Just to confirm the test and give me a little bit more peace of mind. The words that came out of my mouth next, I would regret bitterly for months: "I wish I felt some nausea, you know, just so I would know everything is on track."

Fast-forward two weeks. I was six weeks pregnant, almost exactly. I can't recall what started first – the aversion to food, the heightened sense of smell, or the rumbling, unsettling, sour sensation rising up my throat. It was clear: My call to the universe had been answered! But only partially. I'd asked the universe for TV-style morning sickness. A tickle of nausea first thing in the morning, which would then politely disappear after eating a piece of toast. Instead, what I experienced for the next four months truly felt like a journey to hell and back.

Each day from that point on would bring new misery. I lived not only day to day but hour to hour. There was not a single stretch of time that I could count as rest or downtime from the nausea. My day would begin with feeling ill and tired, and end the same way. Well, not quite the same.

Around 4 pm a new, stronger wave of nausea would settle in. It was all I could do to finish work, scrape myself into the car, and drive home hunched over the wheel with the window open. Once I'd made it home, I'd flick my heels off and slump into bed, dizzy and engulfed by nausea. (Of course, I didn't have this 'luxury' in my second pregnancy – but more on dealing with morning sickness while caring for other children later!) From here I would shun all light and stimuli and essentially writhe away the hours before finally falling asleep. Sleep offered some relief – but not for long. Like clockwork, my body would awaken every two to three hours, forcing me to the bathroom to vomit.

I was throwing up at least three or four times per day, every day. Often, I would have nothing left in my poor overworked stomach but a toxic, yellow substance that re-minded me of concentrated orange juice. The taste alone was enough to send me back into the spiral. For months, the toilet bowl was one of my closest acquaintances. It was a sad, lonely time.

I avoided cooking shows like the plague. Was I crazy or could I smell the meat frying through the TV? Okay, maybe it was a whiff of the neighbours' cooking wafting in the window. Ugh. Any and all smells were off limits. I searched far and wide for fragrance-free soap, shampoo, and deodorant. It felt like I was holding my breath as often as not. Even certain songs made me feel sick. Like Pavlov's dog, even today I can't listen to certain songs from the morning sickness era.

I recall saying to my husband between tears one night, "This is not living. This just *existing*!" I still feel these words completely capture the dilemma of morning sick-ness. Of course, I was delighted to be having a baby. While so many amazing people were struggling with infertility and other serious issues during pregnancy, I was one of the lucky ones... and yet. Always, I held two powerful realities close to my heart – I was so fortunate to be pregnant, and so sick I couldn't enjoy a minute of it.

It was during this time I had my lightbulb moment. I needed to act. Call it survival instinct! Or maybe it was just desperation. But the pure fear of having to continue to flounder around in a swamp of morning sickness motivated me to act. I could no longer continue to just exist.

I knew I couldn't control the fact I had morning sickness. But perhaps I could ease the symptoms. I read a lot during this time. If you've ever tried to read while nauseated, tired, or dizzy, you'll know that's no mean feat! That's why I've made these hacks short and sweet. I want other mamas to learn some hacks without having to trawl through page after page of advice. (Of course, if you are so inclined, I have included additional information, including some fascinating theories on morning sickness, at the beginning.)

I also talked to other women a lot during this time and gained an enormous amount of advice – tips, traps, and everything in between. But the most important thing I gained from this community was a sense of belonging. I was not alone. You are not alone. We've got this! For every Instagram or blog post featuring a fit, healthy mama-to-be practising yoga at 6 am or sitting down to a beautifully balanced, alkaline meal, there are dozens of other women living off a constant stream of potato chips or spending their spare time lying down in a darkened room!

So, armed with a newfound sense of optimism that can only come from a sense of shared experience, I methodically tested every piece of advice and wisdom I could get my hands on. What came next was a journey of ups and downs; of failures and eventual successes. Some of the things that saw me through the lowest points in my morning sickness journey came from the simplest tips, passed on knowingly from family, friends, or sympathetic work colleagues.

Each pregnancy is different, but we come together through the sharing of collective wisdom. We have been doing this for many thousands of years. No two women are exactly alike. What triggers feelings of revulsion in one woman will be another's lifesaving staple. My sister ate a lot of fruit toast in her pregnancy, while I was violently opposed eating any form of fruit. One of the only things I could stomach was rice, but my sister could not cope with the smell or the texture of it whatsoever. So how will you know what may work for you? Trust your instincts, listen to your body, and take a leap of faith.

I have compiled morning sickness hacks with the highest popularity and success rates in the hope that you will find relief, support, and, above all, faith that you too can conquer this all-too-common experience.

Disclaimer

The content provided in this eBook is for informational purposes only and should not be considered a substitute for advice from a healthcare professional. The statements made about specific treatments and products throughout the book are not intended to diagnose, treat, cure, or prevent disease. Please consult with a physician or health professional regarding your individual health and medical condition.

I repeat: If you have any concerns related to your health, see a registered health professional. I am not medically qualified to advise you about your pregnancy or morning sickness symptoms. I am simply a busy mum who has compiled and curated an easy reference list of remedies, tips, and wisdom that have helped other women manage their morning sickness. All hacks are natural and medication-free, and you can do most of them at home for a relatively low cost.

CHAPTER ONE

Introduction

THE TERM 'MORNING SICKNESS' is a farce. Let's start there! Anyone who has experienced pregnancy-related nausea or vomiting knows that it is certainly not restricted to mornings. If only! In fact, many women – like us – find themselves feeling worse at other, seemingly random, times of day. For me, late afternoons and evenings were the absolute worst. And sure enough, research shows that there are good reasons why morning sickness may feel worse later in the day for some women. So, with that in mind, I have included a few useful tips for 'evening sickness' sufferers.

Many definitions of morning sickness emphasise that the condition occurs in the first trimester – that is, the first three months of a woman's pregnancy.[1] Certainly, for many women, symptoms do ease by around the sixteenth week.[2] But for the unlucky remainder (ourselves included), it can continue for many weeks more. Whether it's from morning sickness, an unpleasant bout of food poisoning, or a rough and rolling boat journey, feeling helpless while nausea and vomiting take over is pure misery. That is precisely why I created this book – to provide as many useful hints and hacks as possible to help you through this hellish experience, whether it lasts one trimester or your entire pregnancy.

So if feelings of nausea come at any and all times of day, with no emphasis on the morning, where exactly did the term 'morning sickness' originate? Actually, 'morning sickness' is mentioned in medical journals dating back as early as 1860. Reading that particular article is a hilarious throwback – the author suggests that both champagne and opium are "especially advantageous" treatments![3]

But why has 'morning sickness' as a term for nausea and vomiting in pregnancy endured? It's a difficult question to answer, but it seems to be widely agreed that it probably relates to the fact that low blood sugar and an empty stomach can exacerbate pregnancy nausea.[4] In the morning, when you wake, it may well have been over eight hours since you last ate. Your stomach has been busily digesting your dinner while you have been sleeping, and finally, hours later, your blood sugar levels drop to their lowest level. In defence of the term, certainly most pregnant women do feel some kind of nausea first thing in the morning.

Regardless of how inaccurate the term is, we continue to use it. Why? Well, the main reason is that it's firmly entrenched in the modern vernacular. A simple Google search yields over 73 million results for the term. More recently, though, there has been an effort in medical literature and among the medical community to term the condition more accurately as NVP (Nausea and Vomiting in Pregnancy).[5] Little by little the term is becoming more common in pregnancy blogs and forums. However, it might be a little early to start telling people you have NVP, unless you want to be met with a blank stare!

I have my fingers crossed that NVP will become as widely used an acronym as GERD[6] or IBS[7]. It seems to lend a bit more gravitas to the condition. For the purposes of our book, however, I have stuck with the term 'morning sickness' (even though I agree it is grossly inadequate).

A word on hyperemesis gravidarum

At this point I want to mention that there's something even worse than the misconception that morning sickness means nothing more than a tinge of nausea in the first trimester, and that's lumping *hyperemesis gravidarum* (HG) in the same category. My own sister survived two HG pregnancies and I can tell you that the injustice of the comparison is akin to someone telling you your dislocated shoulder is merely sprained. Alas, the world is full of unfair medical approximations, like calling a migraine a headache or likening endometriosis to period pain.

Hyperemesis gravidarum is a rare, debilitating pregnancy condition marked by rapid weight loss, malnutrition, and dehydration due to unrelenting nausea and/or vomiting, with potential adverse consequences for both the mama-to-be and the newborn(s).[8] The key word here is *unrelenting*. HG is typically associated with:

- extreme nausea, food aversion, and frequent vomiting
- loss of over 5% of pre-pregnancy body weight (usually over 10%)
- dehydration
- nutritional deficiencies
- metabolic imbalances

- difficulty with daily activities.

HG usually extends well beyond the first trimester and, unfortunately, for half of HG sufferers it continues into the third trimester. Complications of vomiting (e.g. gastric ulcers, oesophageal bleeding, malnutrition, etc.) may also contribute to and worsen ongoing nausea.

While many of our hacks are suitable for managing symptoms of HG, our book is not aimed at women suffering from HG. In most cases of HG, medical intervention is necessary and specialist advice should be sought.

For more information and support for HG, please visit these wonderful support sites:

www.hyperemesis.org

www.helpher.org

CHAPTER TWO

What is morning sickness?

MORNING SICKNESS CAN be defined simply as the nausea (which may or may not lead to vomiting) experienced by women during pregnancy.[9] It is extremely common. The signs of morning sickness are very well known by sufferers, but how would I describe it to someone who has not experienced it? Where do I start? Here are some fantastic quotes that go some way to explaining morning sickness.

"It's horrible. Like a hangover without the good time."
— Joni Rodgers

"I started playing poker in 2003 during my pregnancy to distract myself from my awful morning sickness. For months all I did was cry and play Texas Hold'em."
— Cheryl Hines

"Amy is still pregnant and puking because money rarely goes to medical studies for women such as hyperemesis or endometriosis and instead goes to things like d-cks not getting hard enough or old guys who want harder d-cks."
— Amy Schumer (HG sufferer)

"Can't eat because of nausea. Nauseous because I can't eat."
— Unknown

Over the next few chapters, I will explore several theories about what causes morning sickness. As with so many things in life, it appears that morning sickness can't be fully understood with a single theory, but probably comes down to a combination of factors.

CHAPTER THREE

Hormones, baby!

URING PREGNANCY, THE 'big daddy' (or should I say 'mummy') is a hormone called 'human chorionic gonadotrophin' (hCG). It is totally unique to pregnancy.

Your body starts to produce hCG about 11 days after conception, at which point the presence of hCG in your blood can confirm to your doctor that you are in the early stages of pregnancy.[10] Your hCG then increases (roughly doubles) every 72 hours right up until you are about 8–11 weeks pregnant. After this period, hCG levels drop and remain steady until several weeks after your baby arrives.

All your life your body has been functioning with a known array of about 50 hormones.[11] Now, all of a sudden, there is a new one. A hormone that the wise old systems in your body have never seen the likes of before. And it is increasing at an alarming rate! Human chorionic gonadotrophin is thought to be the main culprit behind morning sickness, and when you look at it this way, it's little wonder.

But what about our friends oestrogen and progesterone? Normally your levels of oestrogen and progesterone rise and fall in tune with your cycle, but during pregnancy they remain elevated – again, an uncommon experience for your body to deal with. Progesterone is the hero hormone that maintains your uterine lining before the placenta forms, keeping your baby alive. Oestrogen aids the development of the foetus and later helps ready your breasts for milk production.[12]

So there it is. Case solved! The combination of new and increased hormones causes morning sickness... right?

Not quite.

Many women don't experience morning sickness at all. They're the friends who seem to glow with good health and vitality while you can barely muster the energy to shower. Yet strangely, studies show no significant difference in hormone levels between women with morning sickness and those without. How can this be?

Well, the short answer is that we still don't quite know. Some research suggests that genes may be involved. Interestingly, there are a few studies that show morning sickness prevalence to be lot lower in Asian populations compared to Western countries.[13] And there certainly seems to be a link between hyperemesis gravidarum and genetics.[14] Do you have a relative who experienced heightened symptoms of nausea and vomiting during her pregnancy? Well, according to research conducted at the University of California, you are 17 percent more likely than the average woman to experience the same.[15]

Still, not much is known on the interplay between pregnancy, hormones, and genetics. What is evident is that the onset of morning sickness does coincide with peak levels of hCG.[16]

CHAPTER FOUR

A spoonful of sugar

A WAY TO INCREASE your metabolism without diet or exercise – surely it can't be true? Turns out it is. But there is a catch.

In the early stages of pregnancy, the sheer amount of work it takes to grow a baby (and a placenta) will increase your metabolic rate by around 20%. This means you'll burn though what you eat around 20% faster than before.[17]

For many women, the following scenario is all too familiar. You've been busily working at your desk or churning through housework when you suddenly realise it's been an hour or two since breakfast. Cue awful waves of morning sickness and that gnawing, unpleasant hunger that's so particular to pregnancy. Why are you feeling this way? It's simple: you have burned through (metabolised) your last meal much more quickly than usual, and your blood sugar levels have already begun to fall. Your brain senses something is amiss and triggers the symptoms of morning sickness. It's not doing it just to punish you – it's doing it so that you will act to rectify the situation, to stabilise your blood sugar levels.

If you maintain your usual breakfast/lunch/dinner routine during early pregnancy, your blood sugar levels will swing up and down like a wild roller-coaster. Not exactly ideal. For diabetics, low blood sugar – *hypoglycaemia*, or a 'low' – can be potentially life threatening. But for pregnant women, it's usually just extremely unpleasant! The good news is that to the extent that morning sickness may be related to low blood sugar, it is at least partly preventable. Even just a small snack before you are hungry can help prevent your blood sugar from dropping and stave off an attack of nausea.

CHAPTER FIVE

What's old is new again

ANOTHER POPULAR THEORY about morning sickness attributes the nausea, vomiting, and food aversion experienced in pregnancy to an evolutionary adaptation. Several scientific journals have published studies suggesting that, over thousands of years, women's bodies have developed an extreme sickness response to environmental cues, such as certain foods, in order to prevent potential harm to a foetus.[18]

The theory is that, during pregnancy, you are especially vulnerable to all the nasty bacteria and other germs that may be present in food. Normally your body fights off these pathogens, but when you are pregnant, you have the double whammy of a weakened immune response coupled with potentially devastating effects for your baby if you were to get food poisoning.

But how exactly does feeling ill at the smell of a wholesome roast dinner or gagging at a nutritious veggie salad help anyone? Surely it would be better for both mum and baby if morning sickness didn't exist and you could enjoy a nourishing, varied diet? Well, yes and no. You see, humans have not always lived the way we do now. In fact, even now many people still live in circumstances where there is a high likelihood of exposure to foodborne pathogens.

The key to the evolutionary explanation of morning sickness lies in the types of foods that have been shown, anecdotally and in scientific research, to trigger morning sickness – meat, eggs, poultry, fish, and even vegetables.[19] These same triggers seem to be common to meat-eating cultures across the globe. In some ways, little has changed in thousands of years.

Though we in first-world communities now have access to refrigeration and food sanitation processes that are our ancestors couldn't have dreamed of, meat, eggs, and vegetables still carry a higher risk of contamination for our bodies than, say, a dry cracker. Because these are fresh foods, they are also quick to spoil, which can introduce other microorganisms that might harm a foetus. *Listeria*, for example, can even be fatal to the foetus.[20] Foods that are susceptible to *Listeria* contamination – such as raw seafood, cold meats, eggs, pre-cut salads, and diced fruit – all fall into the above-mentioned categories. I go in to these foods and many more foods to avoid in my next book *"101 mind-boggling things to AVOID during PREGNANCY – The only guide for your inner helicopter parent self"* (visit www.busymama.com.au to find out more.)

So, could avoiding certain foods when pregnant really spell the survival of the human race? Well, research suggests it might just be Mother Nature's way of trying to protect future generations.

CHAPTER SIX

But wait – Is this morning sickness?

D ID I MENTION that morning sickness is a witch with many guises? Most people know about the vomiting and nausea. But fewer know about the other faces of morning sickness. You know, because the feeling of a perpetual tequila hangover combined with an intense revulsion for normal food isn't enough! I have some other delightful symptoms that go hand in hand with morning sickness. How many are you enjoying!?

Sensory aversion

Even women with very mild or few morning sickness symptoms are likely to have the very strange experience of being completely and uncharacteristically turned off by some smells and sights. It can cause such an extreme reaction that is has become the stuff of pregnancy memes and sketch comedy. But for all the humour (for others!) in banishing certain foods from your house or fleeing from the smell of your partner's cologne, it can be a highly unpleasant symptom to live with. Whether it is attributable to evolution, hormones, or even a reminder of previously feeling unwell, the effect is exhausting. Particularly if the list of intolerable smells grows, like it did for us. An ounce of prevention is worth a pound of cure. Effort put into preventing aversions can go a long way to making life easier, which is why I have included several hacks around helping you avoid triggering smells and foods.

Acid reflux

This one is very close to my heart(burn)! Every day, my extreme nausea and vomiting would alternate with acid reflux. It felt as if drain cleaner had been poured down my throat and settled in my chest. I think the worst part was the taste. Each tastebud was coated in a rank, sour flavour that reminded me of spoiled orange juice. I've included a hack on reducing foul mouth tastes – sour, metallic, bitter – to combat this very problem.

Acid reflux is very common in pregnancy. When digestion is working as it should, the food you eat is transformed into a soupy mixture that then continues on its journey to the intestines. Stomach acid, together with digestive enzymes, usually makes light work of this process. Alas, like so many bodily functions, digestive processes tend to go a little haywire during pregnancy. During pregnancy the upward pressure caused by your growing uterus can increase your chances of reflux. Hormones such as progesterone act to slow down digestion and loosen the valves that keep stomach acid where it should be.[21] Digestive juices find their way up the oesophagus, and next thing you know, you're experiencing the fiery repercussions. Stomach acid is strong stuff – it can eat through wood and metal! By the time it travels up your throat it is not quite battery acid level anymore, but for sufferers it can certainly seem just as painful.

Dizziness

Ever wanted to know what it would feel like to sail the seven seas? Sounds nice, doesn't it? But now imagine experiencing a stormy swell on a small boat. It's sounding rather more sickening, isn't it? For some unlucky ladies, morning sickness is entwined with constant feelings of giddiness, tiredness, or faintness. Once again, it's our friend progesterone that's thought to play a starring role in producing these symptoms by acting to relax and dilate blood vessel walls.[22] Increased blood volume and flow is critical for a healthy pregnancy and is visible to us in the changing colour of skin on the nipples and in the road map of veins that are visible on your chest. But the dilation of major blood vessels can reduce blood pressure, which can in turn cause feelings of dizziness and light-headedness. Other reasons for feeling giddy (and not in the new-love kind of way) during pregnancy include low blood sugar levels and dehydration. Later on in your pregnancy, your blood pressure can also drop because of the pressure your uterus puts on major blood vessels. This is particularly true in the third trimester, when it is advised to avoid lying on your back since the increased weight of your uterus and baby can squash a major vein called the vena cava.[23]

Extra saliva

I remember learning about a seminal psychological experiment where each time a bell was jingled a dog would be presented with food. In the end, just the jingle of the bell (with or without food) would be enough to cause the dog to salivate. I would think of this often as I experienced another of the joys of morning sickness – oceans of saliva. I had so much saliva I had a spittoon (a word you wouldn't expect to have to use in this day and age!) next to my bed. Research shows that *ptyalism* (excess production of saliva) is a by-product of not swallowing saliva normally when nauseated.[24] Each day we all produce up to 1.5 litres of saliva, which is quite a lot when you're not able to subconsciously swallow it like normal. There may be some link to acid reflux, too, as stomach acid is known to trigger increased saliva production. In our book I have included hacks to help you deal with the issue of too much saliva, including how to hide this rather embarrassing issue.

CHAPTER SEVEN

Why me?

"**W**HY ME? OR "It's not fair!" you might rightly wail while hunched over a toilet bowl. Morning sickness is a horrendous experience, and it can make you feel very alone at times. This is especially true when you haven't yet shared your pregnancy news and you are pulling out your best acting skills to appear fresh and healthy.

It can feel like every time you scroll through a pregnancy blog or article you're confronted with images of gorgeous big-bellied women described as fit, glowing, zen, or healthful. Meanwhile, you might be better described as sickly, sallow, run-down, and cranky. It is hard not to feel a bit ticked off by your luck. Sure, you could pretend everything is peachy by slapping on some makeup (rosy hues can really counteract the greenness of your face) and taking a filtered Instagram snap – but you just don't have the energy or the care factor. Well, before you throw your phone against a wall to escape all those perfect, puke-free pregnancies, let us reveal the silver lining of social media saturation.

First and foremost, you will find there are many others who share your plight. The internet is the best place to feel that you are not alone in whatever quirks are going on with your body. Nauseous only after midnight on a full moon? Craving a nice big handful of dirt? (Yes, this condition really exists – its medical name is *pica*.) There are many hugely popular pregnancy and motherhood forums around now. Delve a bit deeper and you'll find many groups and threads specifically about morning sickness and other pregnancy ailments. The best thing is that you can either stick to browsing forums, reading and learning from others in similar predicaments, or join in and enjoy a cathartic rant about your symptoms too.

In the not so distant past, morning sickness was something you kept to yourself. It was secret women's business, like menstruation, labour, and breastfeeding. It was taboo, or at least seen as immodest, to discuss these experiences. Sure, women might have spoken in small circles, to family or friends, but outside of their immediate social circles nobody would really have known what was happening. But now? Well, we can see that not only do we ordinary folk have to cope with hardship, but the rich and famous do too. Thanks to a combination of celebrities' need to overshare every detail of their lives on social media and the public's voracious appetite for gossip, we've learned that morning sickness strikes down rich and poor alike! Of course, oversharing has now reached epidemic proportions... but without it we wouldn't know that we share at least one thing in common with royalty and movie stars. Pity it's not their bank account size!

Of all the women to publicise not-so-wonderful pregnancy experiences, none is more famous than Her Royal Highness the Duchess of Cambridge, Kate Middleton. Kate's experience with hyperemesis gravidarum during all three of her pregnancies has served to hugely raise public awareness of the condition. Never before in history has the royal family allowed such open sharing of medical information about a royal pregnancy, and I'm so glad that Kate allowed the world to know about her plight.

Along with Kate, many other successful and famous faces have spoken out about their morning sickness. Among them are actors Gwyneth Paltrow, Amy Schumer, Kate Winslet, Sienna Miller, Angie Harmon, Debra Messing, Mollie Sims, Tia Mowry, and Tori Spelling. Likewise, celebs Kim Kardashian West, Kourtney Kardashian, Chrissy Tiegan, and Beyoncé have all been very open about this less glamorous side of pregnancy.

Does this help you feel any better? Maybe not. But gosh, it's good to know that morning sickness doesn't discriminate.

CHAPTER EIGHT

Change your life, one cracker at a time

MORNING SICKNESS IS not one-size-fits-all. There are a wide range of challenges associated with this side effect of pregnancy. They can be directly related to your personal wellbeing and body, such as exhaustion, anxiety, depression, and weight loss. But they can also be practical, like caring for children, going to work, and sleeping. Our book shares proven tips and techniques for managing such challenges while you are suffering from morning sickness. The hacks I have included cover a range of situations, and there is something for all kinds and severities of morning sickness. To keep it simple, I have labelled our hacks according to the symptoms they help with:

- Nausea
- Vomiting

- Acid reflux and excess saliva
- Dizziness
- Tiredness.

I wanted to put together a book that is easy to follow but also practical. Many of these hacks are food related. Why? Well, for one thing, your feelings about food are probably the thing you notice the most when you are pregnant and have morning sickness. Instinctively you know that you should be eating – not only that but eating better than you ever have – but alas, you aren't able to. Still, this isn't the main reason why I've included such ample food- and eating-related hacks. It's because, in a way, all facets of well-being begin with food. Food is essential to achieving energy and strength. With some energy regained, you are better placed to have a more positive and encouraging mental framework. By achieving small wins on one level, you'll likely see a knock-on effect with the others.

The aim of our book is to help you gain some headway by experiencing success – no matter how small – in managing your morning sickness symptoms. What is the end goal? That's for you decide. Want to lose the negative emotions about pregnancy and embrace your inner warrior woman? Go for it. Or maybe you just want to be able to walk through the supermarket without dry retching. There is no right or wrong reason for reading this book. So let's get started!

CHAPTER NINE

Hacks

Hack 1: Nibble on dry crackers.

Best for: Nausea

Let's get the obvious out of the way! There is a very good reason why dry crackers are our first hack – it works for so many women! Try a few different brands, and once you find your style (are you a salty girl, or do you prefer texture over taste?) you'll realise why nibbling on a humble cracker is the ultimate go-to for the morning sickness (MS) mama.

Hack 2: Eat small meals, often.

Best for: Nausea, dizziness

Eat something small every 45–90 minutes. If, like most MS mamas, you are eating a high-carbohydrate diet, your blood glucose will start to fall around 60 minutes after you eat. With this in mind, beat the clock by eating smaller

amounts more often to ward off further nausea and faintness.

Hack 3: Eat both low-GI and high-GI foods.

Best for: Dizziness

If you find you are feeling quite wobbly, lightheaded, or
dizzy, you may be experiencing a drop in your blood sugar. When diabetics experience hypoglycaemia, they normally turn to a fast-acting carbohydrate to quickly raise
blood sugar – and that's what will work for you too, at
least in the short term. But even better is to help prevent
sudden drops by eating foods with a lower glycaemic index (GI) – that is, foods that release energy into your
bloodstream more gradually.

A great tip is to try eating a small amount of a high-GI
food *together* with a low/moderate-GI food /or very low
sugar food (like avocado) to give your body both an in-
stant hit and a longer-lasting energy source. Here are
some options that are easy to throw together:

- Pasta or potato with cheese
- Cheese or avocado on toast
- Cereal or oats with milk
- Smoothie with berries.

Hack 4: Eat bread!

Best for: Nausea, acid reflux

Bread. Bread. Bread. You may have been limiting it in your diet for years, but the time has come to make peace with bread again.

Find your best friend – from soft, white, and doughy to crunchy French sticks or pillowy Indian naan bread. Bread seems to be one of the magical foods that most MS mamas can tolerate.

Hack 5: Make your go-to foods accessible.

Best for: Nausea

Keep multiple airtight containers of your go-to crackers or nibbles in all the places you normally frequent – in your car, at work, next to your bed, and especially in your handbag. That way you will always have a rescue remedy on hand when nausea strikes.

Hack 6: Set the alarm to eat every few hours.

Best for: Nausea

If your nausea is moderate to severe, set your alarm for every couple of hours through the night so you can wake up to quickly eat or drink something you can tolerate, like a digestible biscuit or piece of cheese. This will significantly improve your chances of waking up without low blood sugar and morning nausea.

Hack 7: Get some fresh air.

Best for: Nausea

Cool, fresh air works wonders on nausea. The age-old advice to 'get some fresh air' when you're feeling a bit sick is popular because it really does work. Go outside whenever you can. Take the opportunity to get as much fresh air on weekends as possible. Try taking a walk after dinner at night – it will help your digestion and should help you sleep better too.

Hack 8: Relax with a cup of peppermint tea.

Best for: Nausea

Tea made from mint leaves is used globally as a remedy for morning sickness and is known for its digestive calming properties. Sipping peppermint tea after meals is especially popular. Buy a recognised brand so you can be sure that it contains safe, approved amounts of the herb.

Hack 9: Increase your exposure to negative ions.

Best for: Nausea

Negative ions are molecules found in the atmosphere around evaporating water. Think beaches, rivers, waterfalls, and any outdoor areas after a storm. There is substantial research on the health benefits of negative ions – they are said have a powerful effect in improving wellbeing, energy levels, concentration, and sleep.[25] This could explain the rejuvenating effect of spending time by the ocean or a running river. If you can't get out near natural sources, create your own indoor atmosphere by having a tepid shower and staying in the bathroom afterwards to soak up the negatively charged air.

Hack 10: Eat slowly.

Best for: Vomiting, acid reflux

Eat very, very slowly. Have you ever watched babies or young toddlers eat? How about the elderly? There are huge similarities in the way they go about eating. Often, they will eat slowly, take breaks, and dissect food (by hand or using cutlery) into smaller, more digestible portions. This instinctive behaviour makes a lot of sense if your digestive capabilities are not at optimum, healthy adult levels. So if you're feeling a bit compromised on this front, do as your baby would do and eat mindfully – slow down, take breaks, and nibble rather than inhale!

Hack 11: Keep a triggers diary.

Best for: Nausea, vomiting, acid reflux

Jotting down what you ate or didn't eat versus how you felt that day will soon isolate any trigger foods or behaviours that are actually making you feel worse. Even a couple of notes on your phone can help you make those vital connections.

Hack 12: Take your vitamins with food.

Best for: Nausea, vomiting

Are your prenatal vitamins making you feel even sicker? For some people, a surge of vitamins entering the body all at once can trigger nausea. Try taking your prenatal vitamin half an hour after a snack or meal to lessen the impact on the stomach. If you are really struggling to hold down prenatal vitamins speak to your medical provider about your options such as folate only formulations and other delivery methods like intravenous vitamin infusions.

Hack 13: Always have a water bottle by your side.

Best for: Nausea

Carry a good-quality, BPA-free water bottle everywhere. Just a little sip of cold water can really help when you are feeling sick – plus, if you are vomiting a lot, you will need to rehydrate often. If, like a lot of women with severe morning sickness, you cannot tolerate the taste of water, add some lemon, herbal tea, or even a small amount of cordial. While nothing beats plain water, if the alternative is dehydration, add any taste that appeals!

Hack 14: Avoid cheap makeup.

Best for: Vomiting

Bending over while throwing up may cause a runny nose and teary eyes, which can quickly leave you with the dreaded panda eyes. Consider investing in good water-proof makeup – or forgoing mascara altogether!

Hack 15: Ask your pharmacist about liquid vitamins.

Best for: Vomiting

Can't seems to swallow your vitamins easily? There are a range of liquid drop formulations available now which are much more palatable and easier to add to drinks. Staggering the prescribed dose at a few intervals during the day may reduce the nausea triggering surge and lessen side effects substantially.

Hack 16: Eat and drink ginger.

Best for: Nausea, vomiting

Ginger has long been used as a powerful antidote for nausea. Fresh ginger is the most potent form. You can add this to tea and even biscuits. Gingerol, the active ingredient in ginger (the part that gives it that characteristic spicy flavour) degrades quite quickly, so for maximum potency consume it within a day or two.

Hack 17: Carry a wedge of lemon.

Best for: Nausea

A great way to stave off nausea is to carry a piece of fresh lemon (or lime) in a resealable plastic lunch bag. A quick sniff when you're feeling a bit 'green in the gills' can make you feel instantly fresher. A lick of lemon can also cut through the greasy mouth taste so common in morning sickness.

Hack 18: Hold an ice pack on your neck

A wonderful hack which athletes use to reduce exercise related nausea or over heating from exercise, is to apply an ice pack or cold compress at the back of the neck below your hairline. The cooling effect is delightful, and it really does help to distract from rising nausea.

Hack 19: Avoid your favourite foods when you are feeling sick.

Best for: Nausea

Most of our hacks for morning sickness are here to help you right now, but a very simple trick that will reap rewards in the future is to avoid your favourite meals and cooking styles when you are at your sickest. A psychological phenomenon called conditioned taste aversion means we are wired to make associations between the foods we eat or smell when we are feeling sick and the sick feeling itself.[26] It's one of the oldest survival mechanisms we have, and it's very difficult to overcome!

Hack 20: Don't drink water during meals.

Best for: Nausea, vomiting, acid reflux

Try to drink water or other liquids at least half an hour before or after eating. Gulping down water when eating may exacerbate feelings of digestive discomfort. Instead, hydrate yourself between snacks and meals.

Hack 21: Make an acupuncture appointment.

Best for: All morning sickness symptoms

Acupuncture for morning sickness is used widely in Eastern and Chinese medicine, but it is also slowly gaining traction in Australia. In fact, acupuncture is included in some Australian IVF protocols.[27] While it can be easy to dismiss alternative medicine, when you are suffering morning sickness you may just find yourself open to trying new treatments! Acupuncture, when carried out by a registered practitioner, involves stimulating specific points on your body. Many women report that this can help ease feelings of nausea and even reduce vomiting. Many health insurance policies now cover acupuncture, so be sure to check whether you're eligible for a rebate.

Hack 22: Hydrate, hydrate, hydrate.

Best for: Acid reflux

Staying properly hydrated is vital to maintaining healthy amounts of mucus in your mouth, your throat, and your digestive system.[28] When you are dehydrated, your natural lubrication and protection against acid reflux is reduced, exacerbating the burning sensation.

Hack 23: Carry a fan with you.

Best for: Vomiting

Your nervous system can react to make you sweat when you throw up, so get yourself an old-fashioned hand fan from a discount shop and pop it in your handbag for times of need.

Hack 24: Avoid heaters.

Best for: Nausea

Stay away from hot heaters blowing in your face. It only seems to make morning sickness feel worse. Opt for cool air flow whenever possible. Open your car window, go outside often, and try using a small desk fan at work or home.

Hack 25: Consume more magnesium.

Best for: Nausea

Many MS mamas swear by magnesium supplementation for relief. There are a variety of supplements and even topical sprays available to increase your intake of this naturally occurring mineral. But for a budget option, snack on pumpkin seeds (a handful a day provides most of your daily quota) or relax into a soothing Epsom salt bath. Be aware that while oral magnesium supplementation is proven to be effective, it remains unclear whether enough magnesium is absorbed through the skin to meet your needs during pregnancy.[29]

Hack 26: Lean left after eating.

Best for: Vomiting, acid reflux

If fatigue means you simply must lay down after eating, try propping yourself up with pillows and leaning towards your left side. Why? The tadpole shape of the stomach means leaning left can assist food flow through to the small intestine and may even reduce acid reflux.[30]

Hack 27: Suck on a sweet.

Best for: Excess saliva

Deal with your excess saliva by sucking on a hard-boiled sweet. This won't reduce your saliva, but it will make it a lot nicer to swallow in gulps.

Hack 28: Use astringents to dry up your saliva.

Best for: Excess saliva

Want to help dry up your saliva temporarily? Use the mechanics of so-called astringent foods, which cause a dry, puckering feel in the mouth. Foods with natural astringency include tea, very cold water, quince, persimmon, green banana, and cranberries.

Hack 29: Spit into a bottle.

Best for: Excess saliva

Try carrying around a non-transparent drink bottle to collect your excess saliva in. With some sleight of hand, no one will know you are spitting rather than drinking. Trust us, it's better than a spittoon!

Hack 30: Rinse, don't brush, after vomiting.

Best for: Vomiting

Future-proof by remembering to always rinse your mouth with water straight after throwing up. Don't brush your teeth straight away, as this can damage your tooth enamel.[31]

Hack 31: Make a survival kit.

Best for: Nausea, vomiting

When you feel the first effects of morning sickness arrive, make yourself a handy survival kit that you can take with you everywhere. You might include:

- Chewing gum or breath spray
- Wet wipes
- Tissues
- A packet of biscuits/sweets
- Sick bag/plastic bag

Hack 32: Shield triggering smells with a scarf.

Best for: Nausea, vomiting

If you know you are going to face an onslaught of nausea-triggering smells somewhere like a supermarket, wear a large floaty scarf, maybe lightly scented with something you are able to withstand. When you need to, wrap the scarf over the bottom half of your face. Sure, you might look a bit Lawrence of Arabia, but it's worth it!

Hack 33: Practise yoga.

Best for: Nausea

Some yoga moves are said to relieve morning sickness. Try poses that lift the diaphragm upwards, such as Reclining Hero and Cobbler's Pose.

Hack 34: Eat sherbet.

Best for: Nausea

Stave off nausea by eating sherbet. It really is a surprisingly palatable snack! You can even save some cash by making your own with icing sugar, citric acid crystals, and bicarbonate soda.

Hack 35: Carry a sick bag.

Best for: Vomiting

You never know when you might be caught out with a vomiting attack away from a bathroom. Keep a couple of wax bags handy. Likewise, in the car, a large cylinder

Tupperware container with a lid can be a lifesaver until you get home.

Hack 36: Rest on a neck pillow before you drive home.

Best for: Tiredness

Feeling drained and tired after a work shift? Do as many night shift workers do – pack a travel neck pillow and give yourself a little rest before driving home. Most travel pillows can be squashed smaller, and they can prove handy for the train or bus commute too.

Hack 37: Flick off the TV.

Best for: Vomiting, nausea

A curious yet surprisingly common trigger for nausea is the flickering of lights. This most often comes from a TV, but even sunlight through trees can sometimes be a trigger for the most sensitive among us. Thanks to a phenomenon called *flickering vertigo*, strobing light can cause discomfort headaches, nausea, and vomiting in some people.[32] You can easily avoid these light triggers by surrounding yourself with more constant light sources and listening to music or an audiobook instead of watching TV.

Hack 38: Try Tamarind.

Best for: Vomiting, nausea

Over the world for generations women have eaten Tamarind to alleviate morning sickness. You could suck the pulp directly from the fruit but if the unusual sour flavour is a bit strong boil up a small portion of pulp in water, add some sugar to flavour and cool the mixture. Sip throughout the day for nausea relief. Remember to not overindulge in Tamarind in excess has a laxative effect.

Hack 39: Stay out of the bedroom when you're feeling sick.

Best for: Nausea

Try not to spend too much time in your bedroom when you're feeling sick. You don't want to have your sanctuary marred with powerful negative associations when you do finally feel better.

Hack 40: Eat icy poles or suck on ice cubes.

Best for: Nausea, excess saliva

Icy poles, which are so helpful for children with gastro, are brilliant for easing nausea and flavouring your excess saliva. They are also an excellent alternative when you can't stomach plain water. Likewise sucking on ice cubes or chewing ice (crunch) provides a sensory escape from nausea inducing tastes and keeps you hydrated too.

Hack 41: Smile when you think you're about to vomit.

Best for: Nausea

Did you know that a drop in the mouth is one of the body's cues that vomiting is about to occur? Smiling can quickly counteract a gag reflex and may help you stop a puke in its tracks. This tip comes courtesy of the grim world of morgue workers and crime scene investigators (yikes!).

Hack 42: Suck on something sour.

Best for: Nausea

Sour lollipops and sweets are especially good for their potent astringency and mouth-puckering effect, which can really help mask nausea – and give a little sugar rush to boot.

Hack 43: Use natural cleaners on your toilet.

Best for: Vomiting

For cleaning the toilet (a job best left for a helpful householder!), try baking soda and vinegar. The fizziness cleans away any gross bits, and the best part is that it's natural, odour reducing and cheap.

Hack 44: Use fragrance-free products.

Best for: Nausea

As soon as the first hint of morning sickness sets in, make the swap immediately to scent-free products for washing, showering, and deodorising. You'll spare yourself from being triggered by strong smells, and you won't end up associating your favourite perfume with feeling like hell! Many products now have fragrance-free versions, but if you can't find something that suits you, try natural alternatives such as crystal deodorant or even homemade clay shampoo.

Hack 45: Use the Pushan mudra (hand yoga).

Best for: Nausea

Hand yoga / gestures called *mudras* have been used for centuries in India to effect a variety of health benefits through the flow of energy. For nausea, the Pushan mudra is thought to be the most helpful. Hold this pose for five minutes several times per day. With your right hand, touch the tips of the index and middle fingers to the thumb. With your left hand, touch the tips of the middle and ring fingers to the thumb.

Hack 46: Try odour reducing filters.

Best for: Nausea

Amongst the best-selling items on Amazon are odour filters for shoes. Yes indeed foot odour is something most people want to eliminate. But what if almost every smell makes you feel like gagging? Get your sensitive sniffer one of these charcoal pockets immediately – hand it in the car, near your desk or keep on handy in your handbag. You can buy the same thing in mask form too. If you baulk at buying something you could easily make – use coconut husk which you can buy from most pet shops (I'm a hermit crab mum so I know this) and put in a sock. It is a natural, safe and cheap, renewable odour eater. Yay!

Hack 47: Try an acupressure band.

Best for: Nausea

Acupressure of a specific pressure point in the wrist can be used to help alleviate nausea. That's the principle behind wrist bands for flying, and studies suggest it is also effective for morning sickness.[33] If you want to try before you buy, do an at-home acupressure experiment. The pressure point can be found on your inner arm, right between the tendons about 5 cm from your wrist crease. Apply pressure with your thumb for five minutes to relieve nausea.

Hack 48: Absorb kitchen smells with bicarbonate soda.

Best for: Nausea

Your kitchen can be a minefield of nausea-inducing smells. Absorb strong smells in the pantry or fridge with an open packet of bicarbonate soda. It will suck in the strong smells of meat, garlic, onion, or whatever else is nearby.

Hack 49: Up the protein in your meals.

For many MS mamas, getting enough protein is a real challenge. Meat – the thought of it, the smell of it, and the texture of it – repels even the most devout carnivores. But many mums report that swapping to a high-protein diet dramatically improved their morning sickness. So if meat just doesn't fit the bill right now, try other high-protein foods, such as tempeh, edamame, quinoa, or chia seeds.

Hack 50: Chew gum.

Best for: Acid reflux

For heartburn or acid reflux, try chewing some gum. This stimulates saliva production, which can help neutralise acid. As an added bonus, gum can be a great palate cleanser too.

Hack 51: Make sure you're getting enough vitamin B6.

Best for: Nausea, vomiting

Vitamin B6 is known to reduce mild to moderate nausea and vomiting. It is often recommended by OBGYNs in combination with other medications. Foods high in vitamin B6 include meat and fish, but also some vegan sources such as potato, sweet potato, and banana.

Hack 52: Drink coconut water.

Best for: Vomiting, acid reflux

Pure coconut water is amazing for its ability to rehydrate you after vomiting, and it is especially good as an acid neutraliser if you are suffering from reflux. Rich in electrolytes, low in sugar, and an excellent source of micronutrients such as magnesium and potassium, coconut is well deserving of its status as Queen of the Health Foods.

Hack 53: Eat papaya.

Best for: Acid reflux

Going past a fruit shop? Try papaya. Many mamas swear by it. Its unique fruit enzymes can help to ease heartburn, indigestion, and even nausea.

Hack 54: Enjoy dairy foods.

Best for: Acid reflux

If you can stomach it, yoghurt and smoothies are great for moderating acid reflux. In fact, a milk-based drink is a great substitute whenever you don't feel up to eating anything solid. Throw in some ice, berries, or banana for a quick, healthy snack.

Hack 55: Get 'sleep divorced.'

Best for: Tiredness

Reserving your bedroom just for you (or having your own bed somewhere else) seems radical, but it can be sooo worth it. Having your own sanctuary to toss, turn, munch on crackers at 4 am, and make countless bathroom trips in solitary peace can pay back in spades. The other bonus is that solitary sleeping allows you to tailor your room conditions perfectly – just the right amounts of lighting, heating, and blankets to make you as comfy as possible. A growing body of research shows that sleeping alone may be beneficial for improved sleep quality – something you'll be needing as you grow your bub.

Hack 56: Sniff essential oils.

Best for: Vomiting

It may seem counterintuitive, as strong odours will cause most morning sickness mums to dry heave, but it's worth noting that some pleasant aromas have been shown to alleviate nausea from motion sickness. Many flight attendants, deckhands, sailors, and the like swear by a subtle sniff of aromatherapy oils, such as peppermint, spearmint, ginger, lemon, or lavender. Just a drop on a grandma hanky is probably enough for most of us. Otherwise mix a drop in Vaseline and rub on your temples for a long lasting but subtle smell.

Hack 57: Try the Emotional Freedom Technique.

Best for: Vomiting

Heard of the Emotional Freedom Technique (EFT)? Well, it might sound and a bit hippy-dippy and, yes, it probably hasn't got the backing of the Australian Medical Association, but it is a gentle and mindful approach to treating nausea and physical pain. Essentially, it involves tapping your finger on certain energy points (or having an EFT practitioner do it for you) while repeating a self-accepting phrase like "even though I feel really sick, I accept I am helping a new life grow."

Hack 58: Listen to pleasant music.

Best for: Nausea

One interesting study found that when people were exposed to pleasant, relaxing music, they reported reduced severity of nausea.[34] Listening to music makes an easy and enjoyable therapy that you can use to relax and divert your attention away from your morning sickness.

Hack 59: Breathe.

Best for: Vomiting

Deep breathing can give amazing relief, not just for labour but also for extreme nausea during pregnancy. Not all that surprising if you're down with your brain anatomy, since the area of the brainstem that controls our breathing also controls our vomit and swallow reflexes. This tried-and-true method involves slow inhalation with the nose and slow exhalation through the mouth, with pauses in between.

Hack 60: Go easy on the apple cider vinegar.

Best for: Vomiting, acid reflux

Apple cider vinegar has many amazing therapeutic applications, from cheap skin toner to natural digestive alkaliser. But think twice if you're in the habit of adding some to your morning water each day. Studies have shown that apple cider vinegar may delay natural emptying of the stomach (something that can be compromised by pregnancy hormones anyway), resulting in nausea, bloating, and reflux symptoms.[35]

Hack 61: Brush your teeth with salt.

Best for: Nausea

Brushing your teeth with salt might sound more like a medieval punishment for naughty children than a morning sickness hack, but many mamas swear by it. Add a small pinch of fine Himalayan salt to your toothbrush and gently brush your teeth and gumline. Rinse well. If you find it too much to brush, perhaps try a small amount of salt on your tongue to gain a similar effect.

Hack 62: Book a spa treatment at lunch.

Best for: Tiredness

Most morning sickness sufferers will agree that one of the only things you feel like doing is sleeping. This hack came from a close friend who was looking for a socially acceptable place to shut her eyes during her lunch break and found that a one-hour foot treatment was the ideal solution. A short nap, combined with the gentle relaxation of having your feet caressed while reclined in a warm dark room, can definitely help ease extreme daytime tiredness.

Hack 63: Wear loose-fitting clothing.

Best for: Nausea, vomiting

Wearing tight clothing around your waist and chest is not in the least bit advisable if you are a MS mama. We've found that tight clothes mimic that tense, gripping feeling that appears right when you're about to throw up. So go ahead and swap form-fitting underwear for comfy briefs. And get yourself into a softer cupped bra as soon as possible!

Hack 64: Eat your way through morning sickness.

Best for: Nausea, vomiting

We know! It's one of the most curious feelings of morning sickness. You feel absolutely starving... but can't face the thought of actually eating. It is a weird and cruel phenomenon! The problem is, if you don't eat anything you are likely to feel worse... and worse, and worse. Eating small amounts frequently has so many amazing benefits – maintaining your blood sugar levels, supporting your digestive system, and boosting your appetite, not to mention fulfilling the increased nutritional requirements of pregnancy.

Hack 65: Eat bagels. (You need these in your life!)

Best for: Nausea

As we collected data, one food kept coming up time and time again as something women felt eased their nausea: the humble bagel, more often than not with a smear of cream cheese. Just what is it about this dense chewy bread roll with a hole in the middle that works such miracles? Well, it ticks two common morning sickness craving boxes – it's high in carbohydrates and also has reasonably high salt levels. The unique texture and mild sweet flavour make it very palatable as well. But if it's salt you're craving, remember that this could be an indicator of dehydration. Treat the reason, not just the symptom, by increasing your fluid intake. Drink plenty of water, flavoured water, ice, and tea.

Hack 66: Be the best manager you can be.

Best for: All morning sickness symptoms

An essential ingredient in surviving severe morning sickness is rest. More than any other hack in our book, practising rest and relaxation will pay off in spades. This is a huge ask for many women, as we are often very hands-on in juggling parenting, work commitments, and financial strains. But the time has come to learn how to get things done the 'hands-off' way. Become a manager in your own life. Do less of the busy work and more of the directing. We're talking about delegating housework, letting unnecessary work or commitments fall away, using your sick leave entitlements, taking all offers of assistance or help, and relying on others more than you have ever done. Generally, people will be glad to help you out. Remember, morning sickness is a temporary hurdle. When you come out the other end there will be many opportunities to repay all that generosity.

.

CHAPTER TEN

Conclusion

S OMEWHERE IN THE expanse of modern civilisation, we lost sight of the village. We lost the collective knowledge passed down by women from one generation to the next. At the same time, against a backdrop of Victorian prudery about women's health and a modern culture obsessed with highlighting only the positive aspects of pregnancy and childbirth, the fear, anger, hopelessness and despair of severe morning sickness was continually washed over.

With this book, I set out to provide women with simple, accessible information about managing morning sickness. From my own experience, I knew that there was plenty of information around, and much wisdom to be found in the experiences of other women. The problem was, this information was hidden like precious pearls in an enormous ocean of irrelevant information. Someone needed to sift through the research and trawl the blogs, but also actually listen to what real women were saying about dealing with morning sickness.

This book won't change the pressure on women to celebrate and be grateful for anything and everything to do with pregnancy and childbirth. But it will provide some much-needed, carefully curated information and advice, compiled for easy digestion (yes, pun intended this time!).

I hope you found at least one of my hacks valuable – and hopefully more than just the one. As I said, the key to surviving morning sickness is to celebrate the small wins and build on those. Small wins and improvements will add up and accumulate to change your experience for the better.

Reviews are like gold to authors. If you enjoyed my eBook, help spread the word by rating and leaving a review on **Amazon**.

If you're interested in reading my next book – *"101 mind-boggling things to AVOID during PREGNANCY – The only guide for your inner helicopter parent self"* visit my website busymama.com.au and you'll be the first to know when it comes out.

About the Author

Bridie Bell

Bridie is a mum of two and survivor of severe morning sickness. She enjoys writing about morning sickness, pregnancy, and toddler rearing. As a qualified Human Resources professional, Bridie works with large organisations to improve their culture and performance. A lover of travel, margaritas, and quality time with her husband and family (including her hermit crabs!), Bridie admits to watching bad reality TV and fancies herself as an armchair expert on true crime.

Endnotes

1 https://americanpregnancy.org/pregnancy-health/morning-sickness-during-pregnancy/

2 World Health Organisation

3 'On Morning Sickness: Its Significance as a Symptom.' *British Medical Journal*, Vol. 1, No. 169 (Mar. 24, 1860), pp. 223–225

4 https://www.medicalnewstoday.com/articles/321734.php

5 https://www.ncbi.nlm.nih.gov/pubmed?term=Raymond%20SH. %20A%20survey%20of%20prescribing%20for%20the%20mana gement%20of%20nausea%20and%20vomiting%20in%20pregna ncy%20in%20Australasia.%20Aust%20N%20Z%20J%20Obstet% 20Gynaecol%202013;53(4):358%E2%80%9362.

6 https://www.healthline.com/health/gerd

7 https://www.nhs.uk/conditions/irritable-bowel-syndrome-ibs/

8 http://www.hyperemesis.org/hyperemesis-gravidarum/

9 https://www.mayoclinic.org/diseases-conditions/morning-sickness/ symptoms-causes/syc-20375254

10 https://www.mayocliniclabs.com/test-catalog/Clinical+and +Interpretive/80678

11 Nosek, T. M. (1998). *Essentials of Human Physiology*. Tampa, FL: Gold Standard Multimedia Inc.

12 https://www.parents.com/pregnancy/my-life/emotions/a-cheat-sheet-to-pregnancy-hormones/

13 https://www.ncbi.nlm.nih.gov/pmc/articles/PMC3676933/

14

https://www.sciencedaily.com/releases/2018/03/1803210 90849.htm

15
https://www.sciencedaily.com/releases/2018/03/1803210 90849.htm

16   https://www.ncbi.nlm.nih.gov/pmc/articles/PMC3676933/

17   https://www.livestrong.com/article/446918-does-your-metabolism-speed-up-during-pregnancy/

18   https://www.journals.uchicago.edu/doi/10.1086/58808

19   http://discovermagazine.com/2000/sep/featbiology

20   https://www.foodsafety.gov/blog/listeria_risk.html

21   https://www.parents.com/pregnancy/my-life/emotions/a-cheat-sheet-to-pregnancy-hormones/

22 https://www.medicalnewstoday.com/articles/179633.php

23   https://www.healthline.com/health/pregnancy/sleep-positions

24   https://www.ncbi.nlm.nih.gov/pmc/articles/PMC3364630/

25   Thayer, R. E. (1989). *The Biopsychology of Mood and Arousal.* New York: Oxford University Press

26   https://www.healthline.com/health/taste-aversion

27   https://www.mivf.com.au/about-fertility/how-to-get-pregnant/ complementary-therapies-for-pregnancy

28   https://onlinelibrary.wiley.com/doi/abs/10.1046/j.1440-172X.2003.00425.x

29   https://www.ncbi.nlm.nih.gov/pmc/articles/PMC5579607/

30   https://onlinelibrary.wiley.com/doi/full/10.1046/j.1365-2036.1999. 00587.x

31   https://www.rdhmag.com/patient-care/rinses-pastes/article/ 16405982/preventing-dental-erosion-in-the-pregnant-patient

32   https://vestibular.org/news/11-21-2013/lighting-flicker-health-concerns

33   https://www.ncbi.nlm.nih.gov/pubmed/18243942

34
https://www.sciencedirect.com/science/article/pii/S00036 8701300149X

35   https://www.ncbi.nlm.nih.gov/pmc/articles/PMC2245945/